Sweaty Hugs

How Free Fitness Is Changing Lives

Kathleen Anderson

Published by Sweaty Hugs
Edinburgh, Scotland
sweatyhugsthebook@gmail.com
www.sweatyhugsthebook.com

First published by Sweaty Hugs, 2017

Cover art & design by Kristen Mann
Photography by Diana Hunt

A catalogue record for this book is available from the British Library.

ISBN: 9781910829219

Printed and bound by Bell and Bain Ltd, Glasgow.

Contents

Contents

Introduction

When I first moved to the United States, fitness was never something I thought would be a part of my experience, let alone become one of the most significant and important aspects of my life there. I think I was so worried about what I had gotten myself into by moving to a different country on my own that I hadn't actually thought about what I was going to do on a daily basis once I arrived. Yet two years later, here we are. Fitness is now one of the most significant aspects of my life and something that helped me find my community in Boston. All because I found a free grassroots fitness movement in Boston called "November Project."

When I first joined November Project, I thought I would never become one of those people whose entire social media is overrun with November Project pictures, posts, tweets, and snaps. I used to untag pictures and had only one shirt branded with the November Project signature spray-painted logo. But recently I looked at my Facebook page and realized I had become that person. I am fully hooked, or as they say at November Project, "I drank the

Kool-Aid." This got me thinking about what a significant part of my life November Project has become. It is not just about working out anymore; it is my social group, my community, and my coach all wrapped into one. And I'm not the only one—free fitness movements are changing lives, not only through physical health but also through mental well-being, support networks, and improved happiness.

This book not only will tell my story of how free fitness has changed my life but also will investigate how free fitness is changing thousands of lives across the country using the November Project movement as a case study. In a recent interview, November Project Boston coleader Chris Capozzi said, "Every person you talk to that comes here as a core member says it has changed their lives and made their lives better." I know I am living proof of this, but I wanted to learn more from other members about the different ways in which it has changed lives. To gather opinions and feedback, I distributed a ten-question survey that was completed by more than one hundred people online. These respondents not only were willing to help me out but also were passionate members of November Project. In addition, I conducted interviews with some of the core members of November Project Boston. You will get glimpses of those interviews throughout this book. I hope that by sharing these, I can demonstrate the ways in which this style of free fitness is changing lives from varying perspectives.

At this point, you may still be sitting there thinking, *Fitness is not for me.*

Well, I hope to prove you wrong!

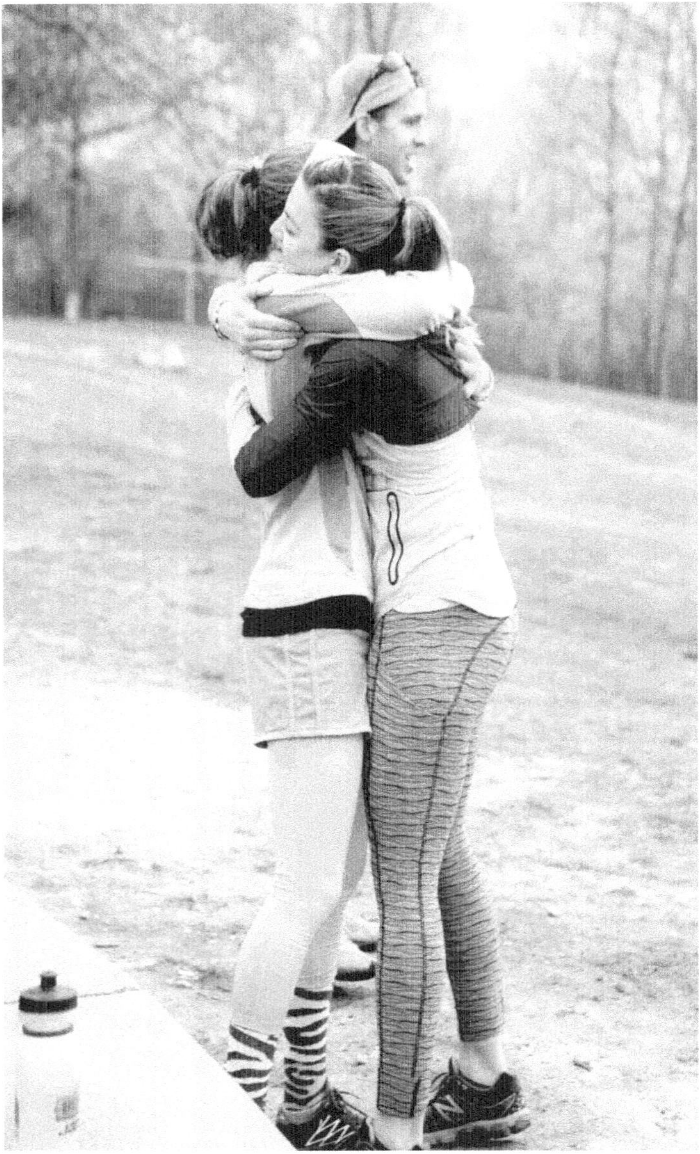

Blog One: My First November Project—May 4, 2015

My alarm went off at 5:20 a.m. At first, I thought about hitting snooze and just going back to sleep, but I didn't. I got out of bed and started putting on my running gear. I say "running gear," but I don't really own much sportswear, so it was more like a pair of yoga pants and a comedy T-shirt. The reason I was up so early is that I was getting ready to go to my first November Project workout. I had no idea what I was getting myself into, but I thought, *Hey, what's there to lose?*

The Monday workout rule states that if the workout location is less than six miles from your home, then you need to run, cycle, or jog there. So I fired up Google Maps, as I still didn't know the city too well, and at 5:50 a.m. I started running. The streets were empty and silent. However, as I got closer to the location, I started to see runners in neon shirts with something sprayed on them. Suddenly, there were lots of runners all going the same way. I hoped they were all involved in this November Project thing, but I still wasn't sure. I then turned a corner, and there were at least one hundred people there, and more and more people just kept coming. I couldn't believe it—all these people looked so happy, and it was still only 6:19 a.m., a far cry from what people at home were like at this time in the morning. Once I reached the group, I got the courage to speak to a girl named AJ, who vaguely explained the workout to me.

Fuck Yeah

They started with a warm-up, which consisted of a lot of jumping, a lot of hugging sweaty strangers, and the chanting of "fuck yeah!" After we chanted this, we had to hug three people around us. I was quickly told that they hug at November Project instead of shaking hands, which can be pretty uncomfortable for a British person. But I rolled with it, as at this point I thought, *I don't have to come back, and I will never see these people again.* Straightaway, I was pointed out as a newbie and was brought into the middle of the circle. They welcomed me by screaming a big "Hi, Kathleen!" (Not embarrassing at all.) Then came the workout. It was tough and sweaty but so much fun. We had sprinting, burpees, squats, lunges, box jumps, wheelbarrows, push-ups, and much more.

One thing I noticed was that they had a great team ethic. If anyone looked like he or she was struggling, then people were cheering the person on and helping. Even though I was a newbie, people were encouraging me and saying hi throughout the workout. It really pushed me to keep going, even though I thought my legs might fall off.

A Feeling of Achievement

Once we had completed the circuits, we ended with some group burpees, which I was called to do in front of everyone. This may have been embarrassing, but it was a good motivation knowing that everyone was watching me. Normally if I go to a gym class, I fall to the back, but at November Project, that is not an option. Once we completed the burpees, everyone was cheering and high-fiving (something that, as a Brit, I always think of being so American!)

The funny thing was that even though the workout was so hard, I had a smile on my face the whole time. It was so much fun, and I felt so proud at the end of it. One of the funniest things happened after the workout was over when I was walking back to my apartment. All of a sudden, a guy shouted down the street, "Good job, Kathleen. Woo!" This was so strange, as I didn't really know anyone in the city yet, but these people were already calling my name down the street. It was the first time I had felt at home. It has been exactly five months since I made the leap of moving my whole life to the States, to a city I had never been to and where I knew no one. Finding a group of people so positive, outgoing, and friendly was such a relief, as I had not yet found "my type of people" in Boston, but at that moment, I thought I might just have that morning. Let's see what Wednesday's November Project has to offer.

Sweaty Hugs

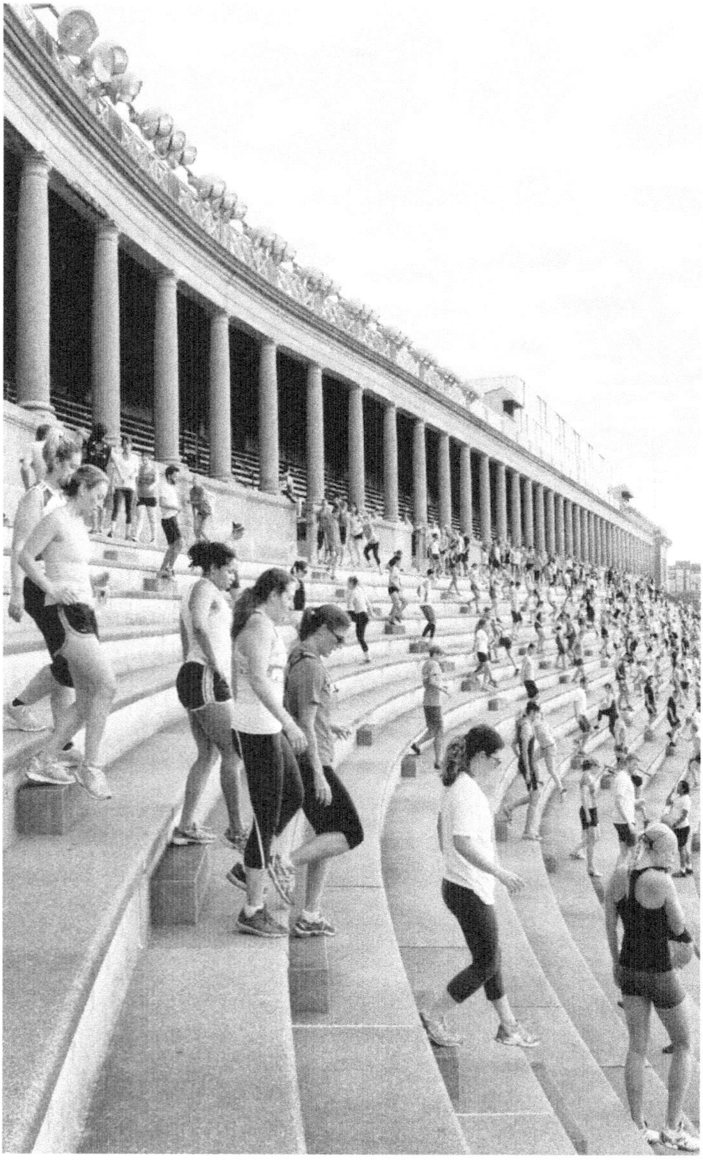

What Is November Project?

November Project is a free grassroots fitness movement that meets at 6:29 a.m.—rain, hail, or shine. In a 2013 article for *Runner's World*, Caleb Daniloff describes it as "part flash mob, part running tribe, and all the rage." At times, it has even been referred to as "a running cult," much to the organization's amusement. The participants consider themselves to be a community that brings people from all walks of life together. It is a movement where strangers become friends and gather to work out around their city. They view the city as their playground. There are no treadmills or indoor gyms involved, and the whole thing is free.

How Did It Start?

In 2011, Brogan Graham and Bojan Mandaric founded November Project. It began as a way for them to motivate each other during the brutally cold winters in Boston. Then they could not have predicted the movement that was about to snowball across the United States. Graham and Mandaric started to invite people to their workouts via social media, and by the end of 2012, on average, they had three hundred people per workout. In spring 2013, two new cities became a part of the November Project family—Madison, Wisconsin, and San Francisco. In December 2013, tribe members and cofounders adorned the cover of *Runner's World* magazine, a turning point for the organization. Today, November Project has "tribes" (each group in November Project is known as a tribe) in thirty states—from zero to thirty in five short years. November Project is a true example of a grassroots movement. November Project employs "a simple sense of accountability to motivate and encourage people of all ages, shapes, sizes and fitness levels to get out of their beds and get moving." Moving may imply everything from walking and running to boot-camp-style workouts. Caleb Daniloff explains in the *Runner's World* article that for everything November Project offers "not a penny is collected. No signatures or e-mail addresses are required. The only dues are good vibes and dedication. And a lot of sweaty bear hugs." The simplest part of November project is how you become a member—you just show up!

In a 2014 TEDx Talk, both Graham and Mandaric discussed the pivotal moment when they realized that November Project had become bigger than they ever could have ever imagined. On April 15, 2013, two bombs went off near the finish line of the Boston Marathon, killing three spectators and wounding more than 260 people. Two days later, more than five hundred people attended the November Project Boston Wednesday morning workout at Harvard Stadium. At the time, this was the highest attendance they had ever had at a workout. November Project had become more than a way to stay fit; it had created a community. People who had never been to November Project before came along because they knew that they would be surrounded by friends they hadn't even met yet, a support group. That day became a respite for people from the press and media that had taken over the city. Whether it was through working out as hard as they could, simply getting a hug from a stranger, or not speaking about the event for one hour, this workout was what the people of Boston needed, and it has continued to be that for many. Graham described November Project as being "a community that people needed." That was when they realized that they wanted to spread this movement not only across the United States but also across the globe, in what they like to call "the world takeover."

Before I started investigating the impact that free fitness has had on participants' lives, I thought that it was first important to establish November Project's objectives. Graham and Mandaric say that the original objective of November Project was to get people up, outside, and moving. However, now that the founders have seen what they can achieve, the core objective is to get people outside and moving *in every state in America and in countries across the globe.* To find out more, I interviewed the coleaders of November Project Boston and asked them to answer what they see as November Project's future. Boston tribe coleader Emily Saul stated this objective clearly:

> I hope that it's this balance of being as everywhere as McDonalds and Planet Fitness but really fucking original, cool and interesting at every single place you go. I want to be able to go to big cities and little cities all around the world, and you find this grassroots feeling tribe that you can go workout with and connect.

A critical element of this "world takeover," as the founders so delightfully call it, is that they do not want to lose the true essence of the movement—namely, community and fitness. As with any brand, the more November Project expands, the more careful they need to be that they do not dilute the brand values. November Project has had offers from multiple well-known sports brands to partner, and they have turned them down or put extreme limitations on what that partnership means. They do not want any sort of corporate associations. The need to maintain this pure ethos is why it is so important that the people who start the next tribes follow clear brand instructions. It's also why the two founders will personally help each new tribe launch, ensuring that it is not compromising the brand ethos. Furthermore, on their website in a section called "How to Start NP?" they have a pledge that outlines just how hard it is to run a November Project tribe and the commitment it requires.

> We know that in order to lead a November Project tribe, will is not enough and that's why we created this application/pledge document that every applicant should fill out to be considered for a position of a tribe leader in his or her city/town.

Finding the right people to help reach this objective will unquestionably be one of November Project's greatest challenges. In many cases, core members of the Boston tribe have relocated and started a tribe in their new cities. In this way, the founders can ensure that their brand identity is not lost. The world takeover November Project cofounders talk about is a possibility, but it must be managed carefully and with passion. In a 2011 video interview for New Balance, cofounder Graham said, "The dream scenario is to be in cities all over the world." Their current marketing efforts have helped them achieve thirty locations. With further development and strategic thought, this rate of growth could continue. But what you will learn in this book is that the true driving force behind this world takeover is the love and passion November Project members exude and share around the world.

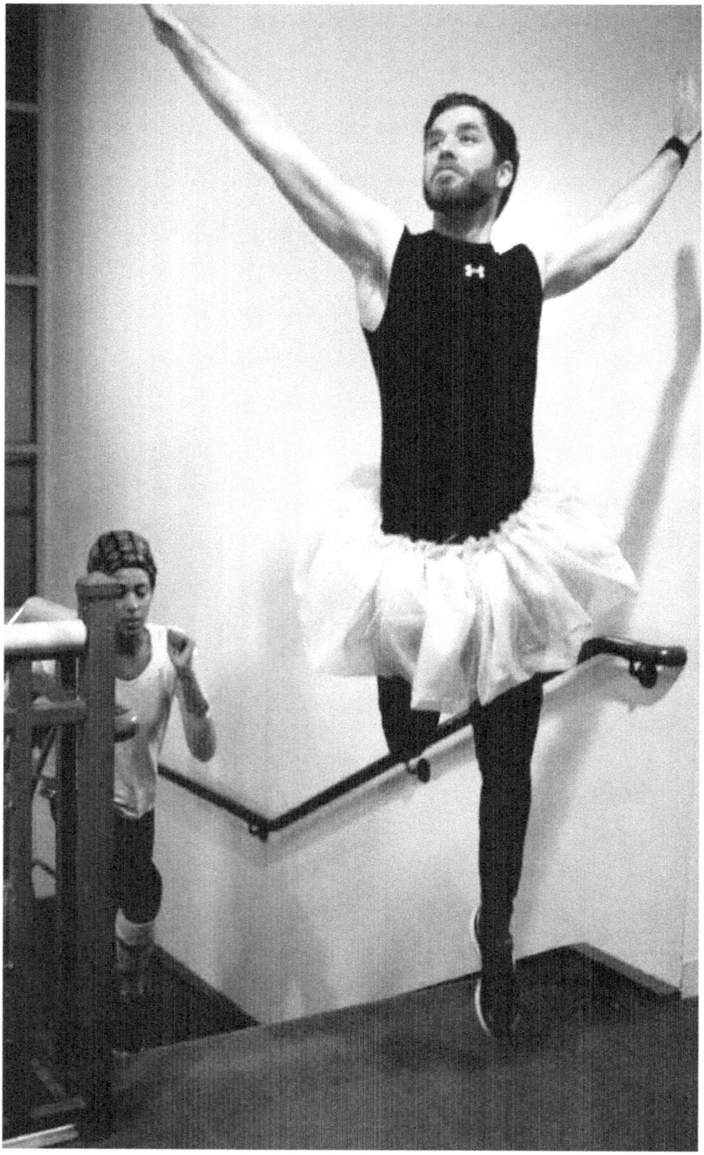

Blog Two: My First Ballet Class—March 2, 2016

Mondays at November Project are always in a different location, and you never know what you're going to be doing. Two weeks ago, we worked out at Boston's famous landmark, the Citgo sign. The next week, we took over the busiest line on the main train system of Boston during rush hour. This week, we were told to wear our tutus and tiaras and meet at 6:15 a.m. little did we know what was about to unfold.

Solo Ballerina

Because the location for today's workout was so close to my apartment, I ran there. With my jeweled hairband on, high bun in, and tutu around my waist, I began my run through the city center of Boston. I thought that at 5:50 a.m. there wouldn't be that many people out on the street, but I was wrong. People were staring at me like I was a crazy person. I even had cars honk their horns at me. I felt like a bit of an idiot, but I like to think that I made someone's morning by giving him or her a laugh.

Usually, as you get closer to the meeting point, you start to see other November Project people dressed just as ridiculously, but much to my embarrassment, I didn't see anyone. Fuck, maybe I was the only one dressed up.

Then I turned the corner and was met with the sight of men, women, and children all dressed like pretty ballerinas at 6:09 a.m. I couldn't help but laugh out loud when I saw my friend, Toby, who was dressed in full black Under Armor clothing but with a pink tutu around his waist. I mean, who wouldn't have a smile on their face upon seeing that first thing in the morning?

Surprise, Surprise!

The workout started like any workout with a little bounce and some "fuck yeahs." But then after some running, we made our way into the Boston Ballet School and were told that we were going to have a ballet class today from real ballerinas! I was so excited because I think that deep down every girl (and guy after the leaping I saw today) dreamed of being a ballet dancer at some point in her life. Today we got the chance to live out that dream.

Less Prima Ballerina, More Sweaty Ballerina

We were divided into two groups. The first group went in for the ballet lesson while the rest of us ran stairs inside the ballet school. Good thing that no one else was in the building, as I think we would have caused havoc in the place. Running five flights of stairs up and down in a tutu is no easy task, especially when the heating in the ballet school appeared to be cranked right up. I have always had this image of ballerinas as these delicate beauties, but now when I think of ballet, I will think of the November Project men sweating buckets while wearing tutus over their workout gear.

Finally, it was our turn for a ballet lesson. We all had to line up at the bars where we were taught first position, some foot-pointing moves, something that looked like a squat but wasn't, some arm movements, and lots of turns that made me feel like I had had a heavy night at The Pour House. (Is it obvious that I didn't pay attention to the professional names of the moves?) But what I did pay attention to was that I could feel muscles working that I didn't know I had. Then—as it is leap day—we learned to leap. Get it? I could not stop laughing as I watched everyone make their best attempt at the graceful leap the ballet dancer had just demonstrated. The prancing I witnessed reminded me of the guys from the movie *Blades of Glory*. The best part about this workout was that it wasn't about how fast you were or how strong you were but about having fun and working out with a smile on your face. I can hands down say that this is the most fun I have ever had at 6:15 a.m. on a Monday morning.

Leap Day

Many people are asking, "What are you going to do with your extra day?" I can say that I spent a morning learning ballet and leaping with the craziest, nicest, most badass people I know and then ran home through the center of Boston wearing a tutu and tiara. Boom, leap day done!

Sweaty Hugs

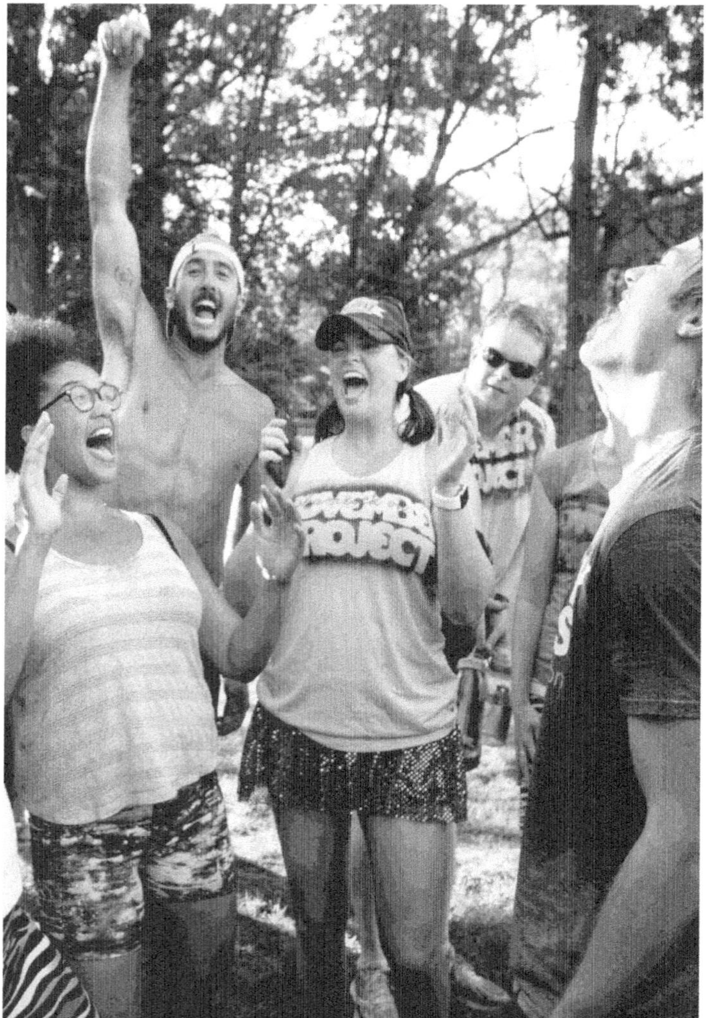

Chapter One—Culture

You're So November Project

November Project has an extremely distinct culture that not only makes it a unique movement but also is a significant reason why the members affiliated with it have such a strong relationship with the organization. Other than the number of tribes that are growing, another aspect November Project views as essential to their success is having a strong and recognizable culture that people want to be a part of. Boston coleader Emily Saul mentioned in a recent interview that the culture is identifiable not only through the "grassroots gear" and the mass workouts in public places but also through the members' energy. She believes you can meet someone and immediately think, *you're so November Project.* She even had people say that exact phrase to her before she joined herself, and I would personally say she is the embodiment of November Project. It is a distinct combination of being a badass but also being kind and thoughtful about the community you are a part of.

But as with any culture, it can take a little getting used to for some. For example, at November Project, you don't shake people's hands when you meet them—you hug. Some people can find this incredibly invasive, but they soon learn to embrace it (no pun intended). Another ingrained aspect of their culture that may not be to everyone's taste is the swearing. There is a lot of swearing.

A key ritual at November Project is the bounce at the beginning of every workout. No matter what tribe you go to across the world, you will start your workout this way. As a gathered group, you start bouncing to get your legs fired up and then the chant. Our coleaders will first shout, "Good morning," to which we all reply, "Good morning." Then comes the question to the group of "Y'all good?" to which everyone replies, "Fuck yeah." For many people, swearing can have negative connotations or can be seen as something they shouldn't do in public. However, at November Project, it is encouraged and embraced as a form of stress relief and a sign of elation. The combination of human contact, comfort, and stress relief can help people feel more connected to those around them and more positive for the rest of the day, as they have started on a high. More than just the hugging and swearing, there are some key aspects that, as a member, you start to realize are an integral part of the dominating and recognizable culture the founders of November Project have established, such as social media, grassroots gear, publicity stunts, and positivity.

That's My New Profile Pic

Social media is how November Project began and is one of the most significant ways in which they spread the word and attract attendees to their workouts. Their members actively tag themselves, like, comment on, and share November Project posts. There are so many people who attend the workouts in summer that you are lucky if you can tag yourself in the group picture from the day. The fact that Facebook even has a limit on the number of people who can be tagged in an image is something I discovered only through joining November Project. Followers engage with the pages and are excited by the content, mainly because they are a part of it. Having such positive content online greatly increases their online reputation and exposure, both of which are extremely important when you have the objective of spreading your movement across the globe. Their social media is not only a way to increase their world takeover but also a big part of the culture. At every workout, people have their phones out taking selfies, coming up with funny hashtags, and connecting via social media with the people they have just met. Many times, there have been social-media contests and challenges among the members. Right now, get out your phone, go on your favorite social-media site, and simply look up November Project, and you will see just how important social media is for November Project.

Matter out of Place

Another integral part of their culture is visibility. Not only through encouraging of members to wear neon clothing and tag it with the November Project logo but also through publicity stunts. It's something that their members take great delight in being a part of. Having workouts in unusual public places not only grabs the attention of passersby on their way to work but also the media. For instance, a few years ago, during one of the famously cold New England winters, November Project Boston members shoveled the driveways of a whole street before anyone was even awake. They not only did something good for the community but also demonstrated to others what this movement is all about. Likewise, two years ago, November Project chose to take advantage of the snow rather than to let it prevent them from promoting themselves. In *Outside Magazine*, it was said that core members "took to the streets of Boston, using large stencils and power-wash machines to imprint the November Project logo onto sidewalks and buildings and plastering cars with fake parking tickets that read "#FREE #GRASSROOTS #RACINGFIT Fuck Yeah, November Project." If that doesn't get your attention on a snowy Monday morning, then I don't know what will.

More recently, on President's Day 2016, the November Project Boston tribe decided to take over the Red Line of the MBTA, much to commuters' delight as sweaty tribe members did triceps dips and squats next to them on the train. The event dominated Boston social media and caught the attention of multiple news channels and sites. In response to the event, coleader Emily Saul said, "We knew if we were ever going to do one indoors, we wanted to make it kind of a stunt. 'Kind of' might be an understatement." It was estimated that more than 150 members took part in the MBTA workout, which even grabbed the attention of T employees, who were not too happy about their mornings being dominated by what many call a "fitness cult." Stunts also encourage members to post on their own social media using specific hashtags and mentions. Again, it's spreading the word of November Project without spending a cent. Members get the chance to show off what they do and share the joy that it brings to them, linking to another key element of November Project's culture—the idea of spreading joy and happiness. I know from being part of the MBTA takeover stunt that I went to work with the biggest smile on my face and took great delight in telling my coworkers what I had been up to while they were still asleep.

Do You Even Wear Neon?

Offline, November Project tribe members are carrying out free marketing for the organization. Every month, tribes offer to "tag" your workout clothing with the November Project logo. Tagging is when November Project participants can bring T-shirts, jackets, and other items to be spray-painted with the November Project logo. November Project-emblazoned clothing (a.k.a. grassroots gear) has become recognizable across states. I can guarantee if you watch a race in any of the thirty cities that November Project is present in, it is more than likely that you will see a runner with the November Project logo proudly emblazoned across his or her chest. This will shortly be followed by a fellow November Project member shouting "fuck yeah" at them. Without any endorsements or incentives, November Project has hundreds of people every day advertising their organization by wearing their grassroots gear. They train wearing it, they post on social media about it, and they voluntarily promote November Project. I initially thought that having your items tagged demonstrates your commitment to the group and shows that you are a dedicated member. However, after speaking to a few core members of the Boston tribe, I found out it meant so much more and is an integral part of the culture.

> I have done it because it shows that I am part of this community. I am proud of what we bring; unconditional support for people of all kinds to get moving; connections with people crossing lines of class, race and the like; helping shape people into highly positive forces in their daily lives and doing it at no additional cost to them, just their ability to just show up and work out with us.
>
> —Elin, forty-two, Puerto Rico

I think of the tag as a symbol of all NP is! Strength, power, community, friendship. Something awesome that has happened as I'm training for [the] Boston [Marathon], is if I am running with the November Project shirt on people automatically start yelling at me in the middle of nowhere words of support and encouragement and love. All because of the shirt I'm wearing with the tag. It is a universal sign of love.

—Kelly, thirty-seven, Massachusetts

I tag my clothing to display my commitment to community through fitness and weirdness and hugs. The tag means community…That tag means I share similar beliefs as 30 other cities. I have a couch to crash on in 30 other cities. I have a running buddy in 30 other cities. I have hugs in 30 other cities.

—Joey, twenty-seven, North Carolina

From these comments, you start to understand that November Project is more than just a fitness group to their members, and they don't wear the clothing just because it looks awesome; it has a much deeper meaning to them. It is a sign that you are truly part of this group and have embraced the culture. These interviews made me realize that November Project has the loyalty and love from members that a corporate brand would pay millions to achieve. When you go running in Nike or Lululemon clothing, it is unlikely that a stranger is going to cheer you on or hug you because of it, but with grassroots gear, members know that even when out exercising on their own they are still part of November Project. I know this even from personal experience of running along the Boston Esplanade and having passersby shouting the November Project favorite phrase of "fuck yeah" at me, giving me that extra boost to run those final few miles.

The Positivity Award

One of the most significant and influential aspects of the November Project has to be their emphasis on positivity.

This doesn't just mean being more positive yourself, but it also means spreading positivity to the people around you and in the community in which you live. I remember in my first week of coming to November Project being amazed at how encouraging and supportive everyone was to one another. When I got to know people better, I found that they had such a zest for life and a positive outlook toward all that they faced. Being a stereotypically cynical Brit, it was hard for me to adapt at first, but I couldn't help but feed off the others around me. Now I find myself being more positive in my day-to-day life. This positivity is contagious, and a couple of the survey respondents agreed.

> Starting days with positivity and movement puts me in a great mood that carries through the rest of the day and gives me a more optimistic approach to stressful situations!

> I have a more positive outlook about everything since joining November Project, which bleeds into giving me the confidence to push myself to do things I previously wouldn't have done.

To encourage and recognize this aspect of the culture, November Project has the Positivity Award, also known as the "PA." It is a sign to all members that you are a true member of November Project in every sense of the word. The award itself is an old rowing handle from the founders, who were college rowers. Each tribe has one and awards it to individuals who do all of the following:

- have a positive vibe and spread it;
- have incredible spirit;
- just show up and kick ass;
- help others kick ass;
- push others to achieve things they never thought they could;
- understand and exude the ethos of November Project;
- are an integral part of the tribe;
- live their lives through the culture of November Project; and
- make others smile.

The PA means a lot to tribe members. Members take it so seriously that some weeks it is not awarded at all. Other members can nominate people to win. I have watched many people be awarded the PA—some cheer, some cry, and some are so overwhelmed that they don't know what to say. To learn what the PA really means, I spoke to a few members about their experience winning it. It turns out that an old rowing handle can have an amazing effect on people's lives.

First, I spoke to Dan, a twenty-seven-year-old physical therapist from Minnesota and active member of the November Project Boston tribe. I wanted to know about the day he received the award and how that felt.

> Emily [Boston coleader] started a story of someone that shows up almost every day, and works hard. She talked about how he had a big heart and looked out for those racing next to him. My interest started to peak and I wanted to know this person. She ended with he had moved to Boston not too long ago and had become a

> motivator in the tribe. Then she announced the winner. I was stunned.
>
> I made my way down still unsure how I had been awarded the PA. I came up to Emily and gave her the biggest hug I could, it all felt surreal. What did I do to earn this? Who did I make an impact on? I couldn't think straight with the joy running through my body. I just gripped the PA and held it above my head and let out a battle cry of excitement and the tribe joined in.

As mentioned, for many, this award means more than just recognition. Dan said,

> It meant that I was doing something right. I had found a balance between working hard and encouraging others so that an impact was being made with those around me. The PA award also made me realize something—I need to work even harder. No longer was I working for myself. I now had others looking up to me or hoping for help in some way. The PA award solidified me

> having more motivation to work for a stronger, happier, dedicated tribe, all running in one rhythm toward the next challenge.

The PA is not only a motivator to win but also encourages the recipient to do even better as he or she is now highlighted as a true November Project person. We then spoke about the meaning to the whole organization of the Positivity Award. We can see it has significant importance to individuals, and Dan made a fantastic point:

> The oar handle symbolizes that if one person does not show up the boat does not hit the water, and if someone is not pulling their weight the boat suffers. The PA shows that this is a person working to make everyone better.

I thought this was such an important observation and outlines a core aspect of the November Project culture—accountability. To become a member, all you have to do is show up, but sometimes just showing up can be difficult. Knowing that other people are counting on you makes it so much easier to get out of your bed at 5:20 a.m. when there is a foot of snow outside. The combination of positivity and accountability creates strong relationships among members and stronger tribes. The Positivity Award is one simple way to award members who are prime examples of people who are not only positive but also accountable.

Next, I spoke to Laura, an author, health coach, and DJ (DJ Phoenix) from Massachusetts. The reason I wanted to speak to Laura was because I have known her to be an integral part of the Boston tribe and was there to watch her receive the Positivity Award for the first time. Many thought she had won it before, as she has such a significant presence, but in fact this was her first time, and it was well deserved. One of the most interesting statements she made during our discussion was that:

> I sometimes worry that because I'm not at every workout, that maybe the leaders don't think of me as quite as much of a "positivity award" type of member of the tribe. I know that's silly, I've been recognized and thanked by the tribe, the

> leaders, and one-on-one for things like DJing or being a good friend, but it's not the same thing as earning the PA itself. It felt good to know that the leaders and the tribe think of me as a positive part of the tribe and someone who makes the tribe what it is by simply being there.

As noted earlier, accountability is a significant factor, but because of real life, some people can't make every workout. That doesn't make them less of a member or less important than the people who do. I think this is exactly the emotion many people face when they are given the Positivity Award, as many of us put ourselves in one box and say that's us, that's what we are. Therefore, to be recognized by everyone in your tribe is of significant importance. Laura then explained why she thinks the Positivity Award is important in the culture of November Project.

> It's always nice to feel recognized for your contributions to a tribe. That's such an important part of belonging: being recognized as an integral part of the group. This is why I think the

> Positivity Award exists. I think we all are important, but sometimes it's hard to see that when you are one of many. So individual recognition for your contributions go a long way in making people feel their value.

The final question I asked Dan and Laura was to sum up the Positivity Award in one word. Laura said "belonging." This has the most significance to me personally, as I moved to the United States on my own, to a city I had never even visited, and through November Project, I found a sense of belonging and a community of my own.

Dan's word was "passion." This is so fitting not only for the Positivity Award but also for the culture of November Project overall. The members are so passionate that they wear the brand across their chests. They are so passionate that they show up—no matter where the workout is—at 6:29 a.m. They are so passionate that they are happy to have every picture on their social media be from November Project. They are so passionate that they will get up early in the morning to cheer other November Project members on at a race that they are not even a part of. The culture has encouraged people to be a part of something bigger than just free fitness. They belong to a passionate and positive community that is changing lives because of it.

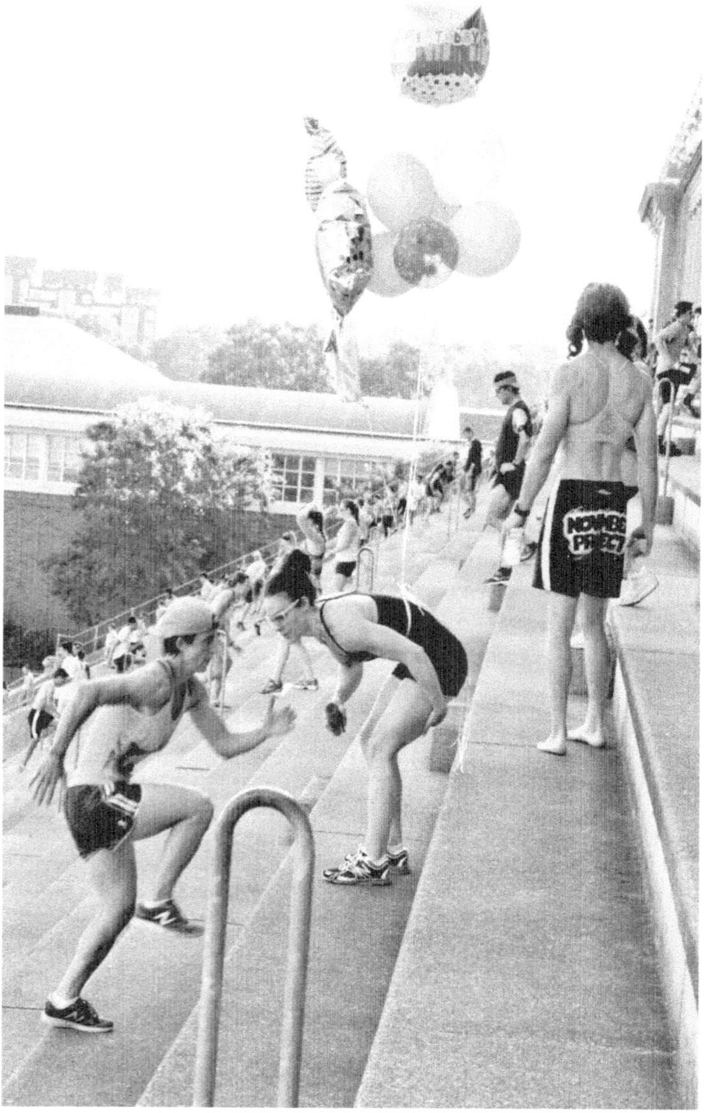

Blog Three: My First Better Than Bedtime - November 10, 2015

Last night, I ran around Boston with more than four hundred people who normally meet up at 6:30 a.m. three times a week. This was my first "Better Than Bedtime" with November Project.

Normally, when you approach section thirty-seven in Harvard Stadium, you would be greeted by a sea of neon, but tonight the theme was black and white, so it was actually hard to see if there were a lot of people there or not. Also, it was 4:55 p.m. on a Sunday, which is not the normal November Project meeting time. But the closer you got—as always—the more you could feel and hear the buzz of the crowd. And there were hugs, so many hugs.

Then came the bounce. We always warm up this way at November Project, but this time we didn't know what was coming next. All we knew was that we were going to do some running. Looking around the crowd, I spotted people dressed as everything from pandas to Michael

Jackson, as this year's theme was black and white. I knew this was going to be a night to remember and something I would never experience again; therefore, I was trying to take in every little detail.

Just Show Up

We ended up running just over four miles around Boston, dodging pedestrians and climbing obstacles. The final destination was "Pop Alston," where a November Project party was waiting for us. We had Harpoon beers, the awesome DJ Phoenix, and lots of dancing. It was amusing being in what I guess you would call a "club" but in sneakers and running gear. Nobody cared what they looked like while dancing; they were just having a blast. I couldn't wipe the smile off my face all night.

Four Years

When I looked at the crowd of people, I couldn't believe that only four years ago November Project was just two guys trying to motivate each other to work out in the winter. Now it is a community of people across twenty-six states—a community of batshit crazy, amazing people. A community that I am now a true part of and that has helped me in so many ways. I hope one day it makes its way to Scotland…fuck yeah!

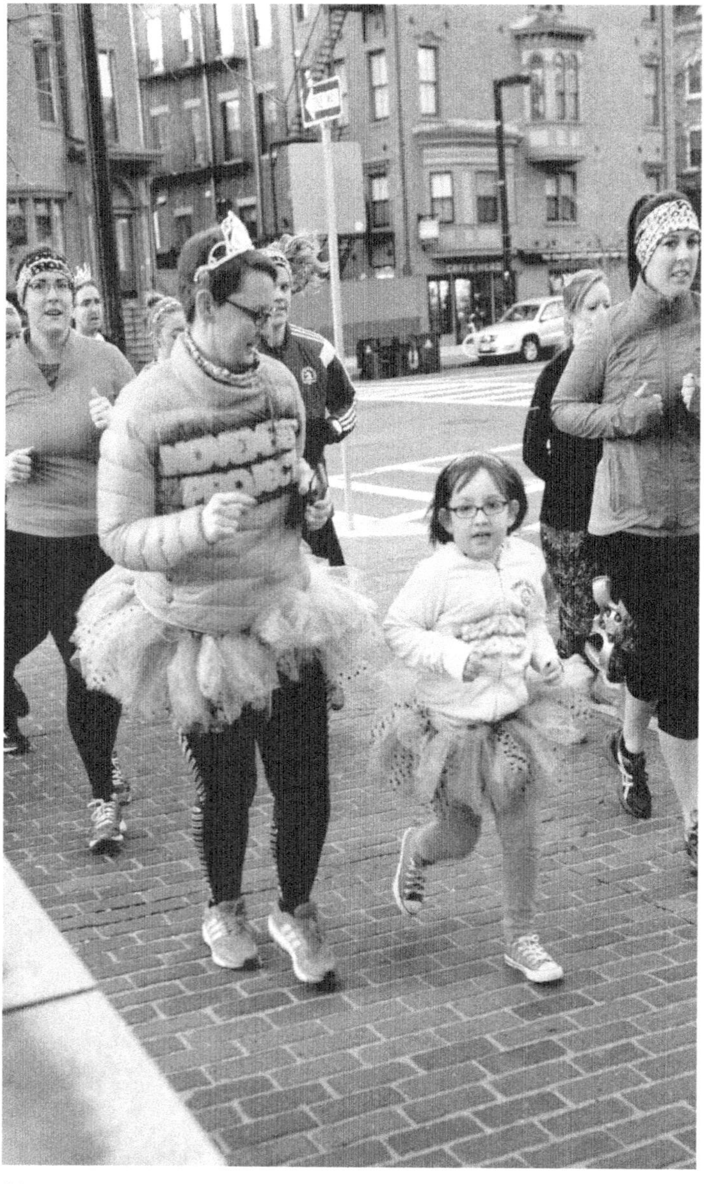

Chapter Two—Community

> I am a part of a community of people who actually really give a shit about each other and the world around us.
>
> —Survey Respondent, 2016

One aspect I believe November Project should be commended for is its sense of community. There are two communities in relation to November Project: the community in which it operates and the community within each group around the world. Through my research, I have not identified any other fitness group or corporation that values community to the level that November Project does. Many other groups of this kind are purely focused on improving your fitness levels or athletic skills. Other groups that have an aspect of accountability differ from November Project, as for many it is about shaming people for not showing up rather than just pushing them to do better. Couple this with November Project's emphasis on giving back to the community, and it is clear something much deeper is going on. It is not just about fitness; it is the movement of social fitness. Many brands offer free workouts, but they are founded on a corporate base rather than on a grassroots base. November Project is never trying to sell a product or a service to you; they simply want you to show up. I would argue that November Project is the first fitness group with a social conscience.

Love Thy Neighbor

> The number one goal and mission of what we're doing is driving people out of bed to get fit and build a better world to live in.
>
> —November Project, 2016

The latter part of the preceding statement is a core objective of November Project—giving back to the communities they are in, spreading positivity and fitness, and making the cities better. Every workout at November Project begins the same—with a warm-up bounce and then hugging. The idea of human contact not only helps spread positivity but also increases the spirit of the group, which in turn spreads throughout individuals' personal communities outside November Project. Some people may find the amount of hugging to be overwhelming, but this is an integral part of November Project culture. The endorphins from exercise and human contact through hugging means members leave the workout and start their days on a positive note, and this can have a ripple effect that hopefully spreads beyond the group.

November Project strives to find creative ways to spread positivity and build community, as sometimes hugging three strangers isn't always enough. A great example of the way in which November Project promoted this objective was in the winter of 2014, when members of the Boston tribe surprised the residents of a street they run on regularly by shoveling their driveways before they had even woken up. *Boston Magazine* said, "Residents were thrilled to find their homes shoveled out and let the group know. In the comments, a resident named Bob says, 'To all you nutty exercisers, thanks for the surprise this morning.' Giving back to the communities in which they operate not only helps benefit the people in that community but also improves relationships between the locals and November Project, as not everyone wants a group of three hundred people running outside their front doors at 6:30 a.m.

Gestures like this have attracted the attention of many Boston publications, further spreading the word of November Project and its emphasis on community building. During my research, I asked participants to state to what degree they believe November Project has helped the community in which they operate through positivity and community action. More than 96 percent of respondents stated that they believe November Project has benefitted the community in which it operates, and to maintain the brand ethos of November Project, they must continue to do this in every city they operate in across the country. However, November Project clearly understands that this is not something they can do alone; it is a group effort. At a nationwide November Project event called NP Summit, Wisconsin coleader Graham described this group effort: "It is now on you to spread how amazing you are to wherever you go…you need to be that ambassador to the next group because we need them to realize how great this is."

Come One and All

The opening statement on the November Project website says,

> Our members vary from Olympic medalists, professional athletes, marathoners, triathletes, current and former collegiate athletes all the way to complete fitness rookies and recent couch potatoes just looking to kick start their healthy life choices. If you think that you're not fit enough to join the group, stop thinking and come see what the fuss is all about.

The founders view November Project as being something that is there for anyone. In a recent interview I conducted with the

November Project Boston coleaders, when asked who their target market was, they said, "We want everyone, but NP isn't for everyone." With their intense workouts, extreme positivity, and emphasis on hugging, it is easy to see why it may not be for everyone. However, what people need to keep in mind is that November Project views themselves as all-encompassing; the age range is anywhere from eighteen to eighty. People may make assumptions when it comes to a fitness group in regard to the type of people who would attend, but your assumptions would be proven wrong with November Project. You are likely to meet people from all walks of life. One way this all-are-welcome idea is possible is the great benefit that there is no sign-up or registration form and no fee. I spoke to long-time member Joey a few months ago, who said,

> There are no "official members." The price to join is participation. The motto of "just show up" does not necessarily make you a badass, an athlete, or even an ambassador. It does mean that you will hug it out with strangers. You will bridge gaps created by social taboo. You will commit to uplifting your peers. We do not do these things because NP requires it, but because it is what good people do.

Joining November Project guarantees that you are going to meet people from all different backgrounds and lifestyles as you would in any other community. But in this community, everyone is committed to supporting one other, something that is not always guaranteed in a community. By removing a fee or application form, you are minimizing the barriers to entry for members and therefore creating a more well-rounded community of people, which allows members the chance to meet people they never would have otherwise.

Finding Your Kind of People

When moving to a new city or country, one of the hardest things can be finding a new social circle. I know this personally, as I moved to Boston when I was twenty-four years old to start my master's degree. I quit my job in the United Kingdom and uprooted my whole life. I was moving from my home where I had great friends and an incredibly supportive family to a city where I knew no one. For the first couple of months, I never quite felt settled, and I remember a friend saying, "Don't worry, you will find your kind of people soon enough." She was right, I did. One way I did was by showing up to a November Project workout where I met some of the most amazing people and made friendships that will last a lifetime. During my research, I asked participants to state the way in which November Project has changed their lives, and there were some phenomenal responses. The following comments are just a few of the profound ways in which November Project has changed the lives of their members:

> It's given me so many of the most important people in my life, and these people have challenged me to push my limits and be a generally nicer person all around.

> I've made so many more friends than anywhere I lived before. I have a family now.

> I met my boyfriend and best friends through November Project. I'm surrounded by athletes who inspire me, and I understand the value of accountability.

November Project, through its tight community, not only created friend groups but also led to people meeting their boyfriends and girlfriends. There are even November Project families. In an era where technology and dating seem to go hand in hand, hearing a story about dating that doesn't begin "so I swiped right" is not only refreshing but also reassuring. The social aspect of November Project and the diverse types of people who join allow members to meet and start relationships in a safe atmosphere, knowing they already have something in common. So next time you think about not going for that run, think again—you never know; you might meet the love of your life.

I'll Be There for You

Community is the true essence of November Project, and I believe it is the reason people have such an affiliation with the November Project brand. Community is at the heart of their success, and helps maintain the grassroots feel (even though they now have over thirty tribes across the globe). Having a community that is supportive of its members was one of the main ways in which survey respondents said November Project had helped them change their lives and continue when they hit adversity in their personal lives. One participant said this:

> NP is a community that focuses on the future, not who I used to be but who I am aiming to be. The members of my tribe have supported me in all of my goals athletic and not. Through this love, compassion and support I have learned to spread it to those around me, tribe member or not.

This statement demonstrates the impact November Project can have not only on the individual but also on people's personal lives, families, and the wider world. The number of responses to the survey that stated that the November Project community had acted as a form of counseling and support for many who are struggling in their personal lives overwhelmed me. One respondent stated that the most important thing he gained from being a member wasn't the increased fitness and faster 5K time but the knowledge that he has "a supportive community to fall back on during both good times and bad." Sometimes all you need in life is the knowledge that someone is thinking about you. Having a community that reaches out to you when you miss a workout and asks you about your life. Simple things that can improve someone's life and help them get through hard times. Knowing that this community is aware of what is going on in your life and cares is so important to the members of November Project, and I believe it is one of the most significant reasons people keep coming to workouts and are so loyal to the November Project brand.

The supportive network that November Project provides has allowed members to thrive personally on many different levels, be it through increasing confidence, successfully battling mental-health issues, or even overcoming a grievance. One participant described the significant impact of being a member of November Project for her was "becoming part of the NP family—such an amazing support system for real-world things like dealing with a miscarriage." I bet no one say that about their local spin class. Having a group of people who will genuinely look out for you and support you in times of need is an essential part of the November Project package. It is not advertised in any of their promotional videos but instead is what you experience after you become a true part of the community. What you give to the community, you get back and more. What follows are some of the statements from participants about community and what it allowed them to do, achieve, and even overcome:

> My participation in NP has made me more outgoing and much less self-conscious. My self-confidence, both personally and athletically, has been considerably enhanced. The people I've met through NP have helped me become more positive and optimistic.

> As a person—I have found it easier to say hi to strangers and offer a hug; I've found it easier to be more positive about myself and more determined about the goals I set.

> Mostly as a person—I've become less socially anxious and more likely to engage with strangers!
>
> I am stronger and more resilient physically and emotionally as a result of being an NP tribe member.

For a fitness organization to have such meaningful impacts on their members is astounding. It's not just about athletic achievements—in fact, they are just the icing on top of the November Project cake. November Project helped me to become a better person on many levels, particularly in terms of positivity. Britain is known for being cynical and slightly negative, or as I like to say, every compliment comes wrapped in an insult. Therefore, I used to think that when people were overly positive they did not mean it, but at November Project, I learned that this is not the case. November Project has changed my life, as I am a much more positive person than I was a few years ago, and I believe this positive attitude has seeped into the rest of my life and is the reason I have been able to accomplish athletic and career achievements I never thought possible. And as you can see, I am not the only one who feels this way.

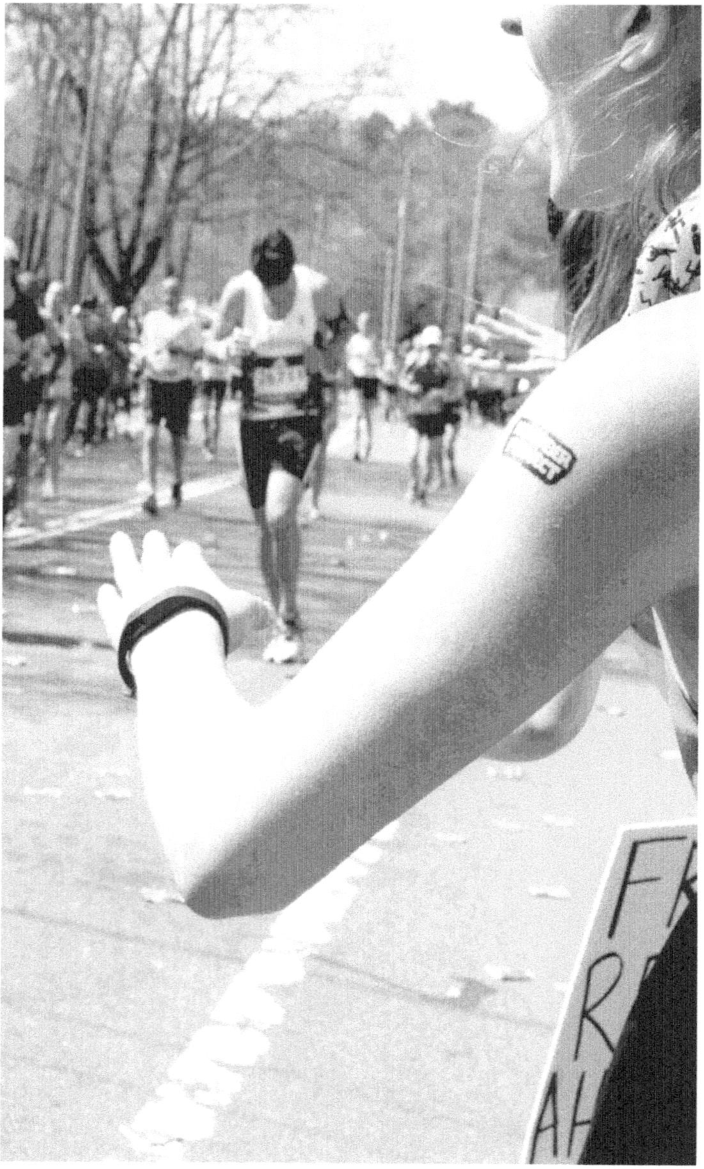

Blog Four: My First Half Marathon—March 5, 2016

For a start, I never for one second thought I would be writing a blog post about doing a half marathon, let alone writing about the fact that I actually finished one.

A Year On

Around this time last year, I ran the St Patrick's Day 5K with my friend, Sarah. It was the first race that I had done in the States, and I found it hard. It was only 3.1 miles, and even then I had to stop and walk for parts of it. I was happy when I crossed the finish line, but the fact that I had to walk really annoyed me and motivated to make sure that next time that didn't happen. That then led me to go along to this thing called November Project, and from that morning on, this running hobby really took off. But even then, the idea of a half marathon was laughable. I did not think I would manage to complete a half marathon a year from then without stopping, and here we are. I guess a lot can change in a year.

Road to Rhode Island

The morning of the half marathon, my alarm went off at 4:30 a.m. after a restless night of panicking about the event. I think I spent most of the night trying to come up with excuses of how to get out of it, which ranged from calling to say I was sick to just staying in bed and hoping no one would notice. But I knew there was a bunch of other November Project people doing it, and they were giving me a lift, so I couldn't back out. At 5:30 a.m., I met the crew that was running, and I was relieved to know that I wasn't the only person doing a half for the first time—this guy Dan was too. I felt comforted that I wasn't alone until he started talking about all the crazy obstacle courses and ultra-races he had done in the past. This guy wasn't kidding around. We were not in the same boat anymore—he was more yacht while I was trailing behind in a dinghy. That's when the panic set in again. I could feel my heart racing, and I started to feel so sick. The whole journey I kept getting waves of nerves, thinking *What the fuck am I doing?*, and trying to figure out a way to get out of it. But having this crazy and lovely bunch of people around me calmed me down slightly.

Freezing Our Balls Off

When we made it to the beach where the race began, we hadn't quite realized how cold it was: negative four degrees Celsius (twenty-five degrees Fahrenheit) with a serious wind-chill. After collecting our numbers and getting our race gear on, we had to wait in the freezing cold. Luckily, our mum (or I should say mom, as I'm in the United States) for the day, Sarah, was there to help us out. She not only let us warm up in her car but also was nice enough to take all our extra layers once the race began. In a way, the cold was good because I was so distracted by how cold it was I wasn't thinking about the fact that I was about to run 13.1 miles. Then we were off…

I swear, the first two miles felt as though I was defrosting. The first four miles went so fast and felt like nothing. At this point, I ran past our November Project cheer crew, and that was so awesome to see and gave me a good boost!

Mind Over Matter

It's funny because I couldn't tell you much about the next nine miles. I know that miles eight to ten were the worst and the time I just couldn't get my legs to move faster. No matter how much I wanted it, they could not go any fucking faster. Then something strange happened. When I saw that ten-mile sign and realized we had only a 5K left, I suddenly got a new boost of energy, and my pace sped up.

The course itself was beautiful, as we were running along the coast and past some of the most amazing houses I have ever seen. However, I wasn't really paying attention to that. Instead, I was thinking about totally random things. The day before the race, I got lots of great advice from November Project members, which included "think about that throwback Thursday pic," "think about the beer at the end," "think about how it will feel when you go over the finish line," "make a list in your head of all the junk food you want to eat after," and even, "come up with the wording for your FB post." I thought about all these things, and it seemed to work. But to be honest, just the motivation that all these people knew I was doing this and had been so encouraging was the best thing that kept me going. Also, I'm incredibly competitive (even with myself), so I'm sure that played a part too.

Photo Finish

I will never forget turning the corner and seeing the finish line. All my November Project people were lined up at the side of the finish line, ready with high-fives and "fuck yeahs." I could not stop smiling, and I started sprinting toward the finish line. I remember seeing everyone standing right at the finish line screaming for me to go faster, and it worked. I did. Once over that line, I immediately grabbed Sarah and hugged her as hard as I could. I couldn't believe it. I think I was in a state of shock as I hugged the rest of the group—so much so that I forgot to grab my medal. I said to everyone after that I felt like I had pulled a muscle in my face I had smiled so hard.

Suddenly, almost instantly, came the pain in my legs, but I didn't care. I was just so fucking happy. It was even kind of emotional, and for someone like me who I know to be dead inside, that is an achievement. After we had gathered the whole team, we headed to the nearest bar to grab some well-deserved pints. And of course, we bumped into another November Project person…you can't get away from them.

Motivational Monday

All day, I didn't feel like I had done it. But then all the messages started flooding in saying congratulations. People I hadn't spoken to in years were congratulating me. And that's when it hit me—this is a big deal. In high school, I was the kind of chubby, unfit girl who hated any kind of exercise. There is no way I would have thought I could have done this, and to be honest, I wouldn't have wanted to. And now I can't wait to do my next one.

One of the best messages I received was from November Project Boston coleader Chris Capozzi, who, when I said it wasn't a big deal, replied,

> It's an amazing achievement! That's the amazing thing about NP there are people that will inspire you to do more but there's an equal amount of people you inspire by your achievement. You should be proud of what you did today, whether it's your fastest 5k, first half or full marathon or a BQ—they are all equally awesome goal! Proud of you!

I mean, come on, is that not the nicest message? It just sums the whole thing up. Without finding November Project, there is no way I would have done this. You have people around you of all shapes and sizes who are badass and make you want to be better, run faster, and train harder. Also, you have this accountability not only to show up but also to crush it. They have helped me change my lifestyle and, more importantly, my mind-set. I no longer look at working out as a chore or something

I resent doing. Instead, it's something I get excited for, and fitness is now a love of mine. And for that I will be eternally grateful!

Sweaty Hugs

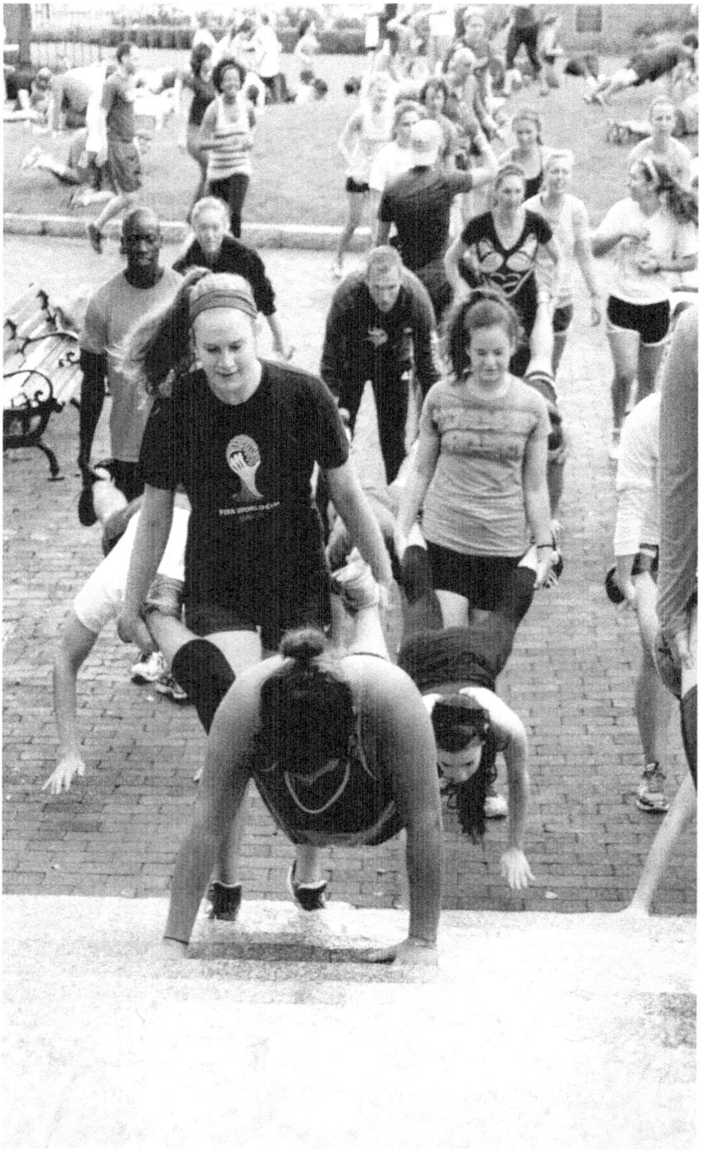

Chapter Three—Fitness and Mind-Set

Push It

November Project was founded on the idea of accountability. Having a group of people supporting and encouraging you is one of the most important ways that members push themselves harder and keep showing up. This can be seen by simply looking for mentions of November Project on social media, as there is a vast amount of blog posts, articles, and social media posts from their members who have achieved something they never thought possible had it not been for November Project. During my research, many participants mentioned the athletic achievements they accomplished, which they believe would not have been possible had it not been for November Project. It ranged from competing their first 5K to running the New York City Marathon in under three hours. One survey respondent said the following:

> Being in NP has allowed me to develop my athleticism and identify as an athlete at all. It's

> made me able to see the results of my determination and made me feel empowered physically in a way I had not been before. Instead of being someone who thought I couldn't run, I now can see I could do just about anything with enough training and determination.

Many people reach these achievements because of the support and encouragement that comes from all the other members around them. I know I would have never been able to do a full tour (this is when you run up and down all thirty-seven sections of Harvard Stadium) if it had not been for my friends at November Project. Having them around makes me accountable, even more so when they are running next to me and cheering me on, which helped me get to the end of all thirty-seven sections. Also, as I mentioned in my blog post, I would not have done a half marathon had it not been for my friend, Sarah, encouraging me and pushing me to train. This is coming from the perspective of someone who is not the fastest person. In fact, I am very much in the lower end of the fitness level of November Project, which is why I found Boston tribe member Selena's story to be so intriguing. Originally from the Netherlands, she too found a community through November Project. In an interview earlier this year, she told me her story.

> After quitting competitive rowing in 2013 I signed up for a gym and went four to five times a week without a goal. So I joined NP in August 2015. At that time I couldn't run long distances because of an injury, but I was willing to do every exercise for that injury to fix it. On the hills and at the stadium, I really liked the fact people are faster than me (in the gym, I was usually the strongest or fittest). I was so surprised how many fit people are members of NP. Every workout I do, I am trying to get fitter to eventually be as fit as these people.

Selena found motivation through people being faster and fitter than her. Being in an environment that not only encourages but also motivates you to be the best version of yourself is something that November Project provides that you can't often find from going to the gym and putting your headphones in on the treadmill. For Selena, it helped her become a better athlete and overcome an injury that could have put her off running. She said that she was motivated by people faster than her, and I can guarantee that for someone at November Project, she was the motivation for someone slower than her. Having peers with all different levels of fitness means that there is always someone looking up to you, and as the tribe is growing so fast, you are never a newbie for too long. The accountability aspect of knowing that someone is motivated by you would encourage anyone to run those hills just a little bit faster each week.

Motivating as Fuck

Although I can see from social media and know people for whom November Project has helped them achieve athletic feats they never thought possible, during my research, I wanted to see just how far this had gone. I believe the most important questions I asked to determine if November Project had helped members to shatter their expectations of themselves were the two penultimate questions, which asked, "Do you believe that November Project has helped you to better yourself as a person and/or athlete?" Respondents were then prompted to explain the reasoning for answering yes. With 97 percent of the respondents stating yes, it appears that November Project is pushing members to be better athletes and people and that being motivated by November Project members was a significant factor in this change.

> People encourage me to push myself and set goals and inspire me to be a better person.
>
> I find I am less likely to give up and to push myself more when I am either at a workout or running with NP people outside of the scheduled workouts. The encouragement motivates me. I am more open to meeting new people as well and I hug more!

November Project was founded on the idea of accountability between two friends. Every morning when they got up in November, they were counting on the other being there, thus motivating them to get out in those cold November mornings. We all know that at the end of a long day we do not want to go to the gym, but if one of our friends is meeting us there, then we have that added motivation that makes us get up and go. This factor is still an integral part of November Project, but instead of just one friend expecting you to show up, you have hundreds. And even better, if you don't show up, then you will have people asking you where you are, meaning you know someone is always thinking about you and missed you. I remember missing a workout because I wasn't feeling well, and even though I had been in the country for less than a year, I had many people message me asking me where I was and asking if I needed anything. I was overwhelmed by this community's support, and it made me not want to miss another workout and to do the same for someone else should they not show up. This appears to be one of the most significant factors in pushing members to do better and to keep showing up and becoming a better athlete.

> If you say you are going to be at a workout, that is called making a verbal, and you stick to it.

> The accountability factor has made me workout more consistently especially during the winter months.
>
> It holds me accountable, inspires me to work hard and to encourage others as well.

Harder, Better, Faster, Stronger

Even though free fitness can change lives in so many different ways, we do not want to forget or diminish the importance of the athletic achievements that occur due to participating in free fitness. Boston tribe coleader Chris Capozzi stated that, for him, one of the most rewarding parts of November Project is when "an individual does more than they ever thought they could or just kind of shatters those sort of limitations that they put on themselves". Chris and the other leaders want new members to join and then perhaps a month or a year from then do something that they have never done before. This could be anything from their first 5K race to a first marathon or even to a full tour. It is clear that this has happened to many members of November Project. The following are just some personal examples I collected during my research of the athletic achievements that have occurred due to being a part of this community and culture of free fitness:

> I found my love of being active again and ran my first marathon!
>
> Well, I wasn't a runner before I started NP, and now I'm training for my fifth and sixth marathons. And I lost thirty pounds. And I'm happier, I have a more diverse friend group, I know my city better, I love running in all weather conditions.
>
> No way would I be running THE Boston Marathon without having found NP this year!

In turn, these athletic achievements lead to health benefits, both physical and mental. I wanted to learn more about emotional benefits of November Project so I spoke to Boston tribe member Erica, thirty-eight, from Massachusetts.

Erica joined November Project Boston in October 2014. She had first heard about November Project on Twitter but was too scared to go along to a workout with the fear that she would be "the slow, fat one." However, she eventually built up the courage and has never looked back. I spoke to Erica about the different ways in which November Project has changed her life.

> I have always felt like I belong in my body when I do something joyful and physical, like dancing, biking, swimming, etc. But basically, November Project kicked that into a whole other level. Dancing and cycling didn't engage me at the level of intensive exercise that NP does. NP has me doing things that previously I had only ever attempted in gym class in school—complete with attendant mocking by the fit jocks. Now the fit jocks are the people cheering me on and taking the time to coach me on technique, sharing my pride in my accomplishments. But literally on a physical level, NP started right away pushing my limits. So being part of NP is sort of an endless unfolding discovery of all the things my body can

do that I hadn't known it could or had assumed weren't ever going to be for me.

Like running a mile. I had only ever attempted that a couple of times. I'd have asthma attacks, and the gym teachers would yell at me and call me lazy, and I would have to struggle through a painful, wheezing mile while the other kids got to go back inside to their next classes. But now, I have run several 5ks, and I plan to run more. My last 5k, I ran the whole way without stepping into a walk. So my sense of what my body can do is just expanding.

I just think that I walk more proudly in the world. That I know I've proven things to myself, that I'm capable of pushing myself farther than I had thought, and that carries with me. Even if some days I'm feeling like a mess in one of the other areas of my life, I know I have it together when it comes to NP. I get myself out of bed and I show up and I work out and push myself and get

> better, so there is always something to be proud of, to be successful at.
>
> I should also talk about mental health. I have depression, always have, and I take meds, but the combination of social plus endorphin highs plus personal empowerment means NP has helped a lot in keeping me on an even keel. When I am dealing with stress in my life, going to NP makes it better. It's the best and most rewarding kind of routine. And someone will give you a hug if you're having a bad week, or celebrate your joy with you, or talk you through something you're anxious about. All the things that a true community does.

Erica's story is one of greatness. She motivates me every time I see her at a workout, yet at first she thought she would be "the slow, fat one." She has conquered mental health, body image, and her own capability. These are all things many of us deal with on a daily basis but don't know how to overcome. She has, and without the help of November Project, she may not have. I think we should all take a page out of Erica's book and stop putting labels on ourselves and just go for those things we never thought possible.

We all put such high expectations on ourselves to be the smartest, the fastest, and the prettiest, and we shouldn't. We need to find a way to shatter those expectations. All the people I spoke to have shattered their expectations of themselves in every aspect, and this is because of free fitness. Having people around them not only motivating them but also making them accountable to show up to the workouts has allowed people to achieve things they never thought possible, thus making them happier people. Personally, I never thought I would run a half marathon, but I did, and I loved it. I would never have done it had it not been for making free fitness a significant aspect of my life.

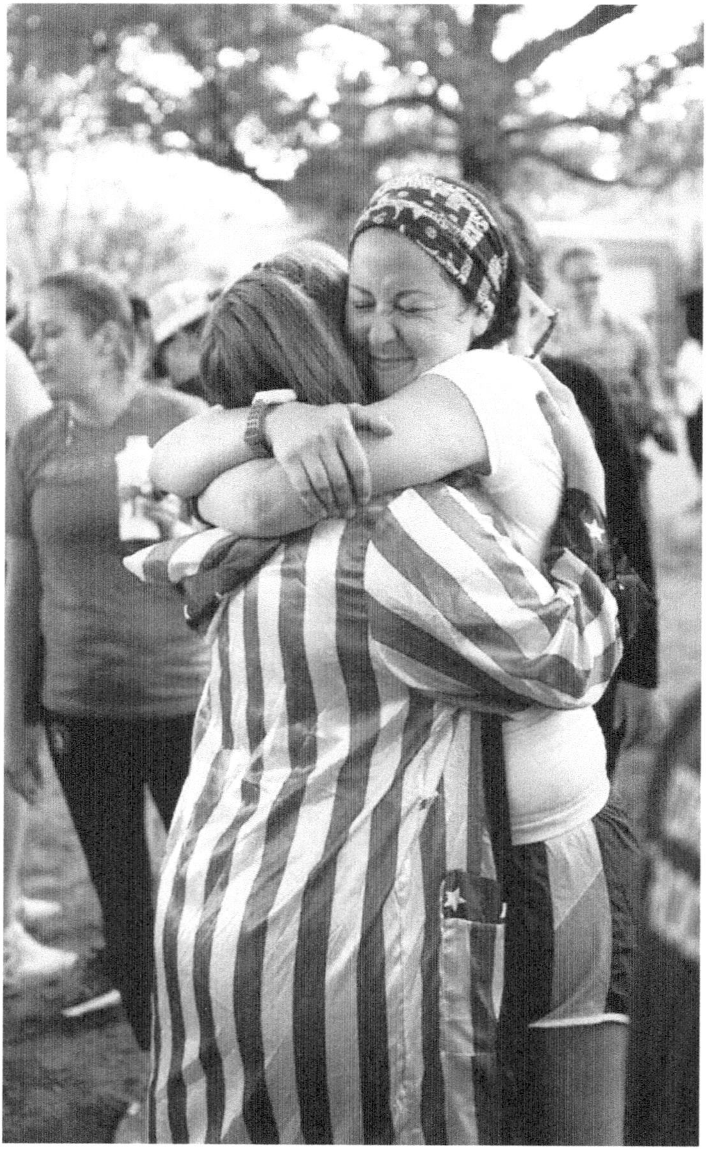

Blog Five: A Year On—January 2, 2016

Sometimes I miss home, especially because I am very close to my family and have the most amazing friends whom I have had by my side for the last twenty-six years. But those feelings of homesickness come and go, and I have learned that they are just part of this whole experience. They say that absence makes the heart grow fonder, and I couldn't agree more. I think people who move away and expect to never feel this way are kidding themselves, but you just have to deal with it, and I can promise you that you will be fine the next day.

Weirdly, one thing that I have found that really helps me is the amazing fitness movement I am a part of called November Project. They are this crazy, lovely bunch of people who I work out with at 6:30 a.m. three times a week. They are my new community, and everyone looks out for one another. They even do big and small things for one another. On days where I really just want to get on a plane back to Scotland, I know that I can go and get a hug from a friend, and I will instantly feel better. Or, if I've had a shitty day and am just mad at the world, then

I know that I can take it out on the stadium by crushing some stairs. I know that no matter what, three times a week, I am going to see the same people, get some hugs, work out in the fresh air, and laugh with people. I believe it would not only help homesickness but also anyone's general mind-set. I know it has made me a more positive and happy person and has given me the chance to meet some of the most amazing and kind people who otherwise I would never have crossed paths with. For that, I am truly grateful to November Project and hope never to lose it as part of my life.

You never know—maybe one day there will be November Project Scotland.

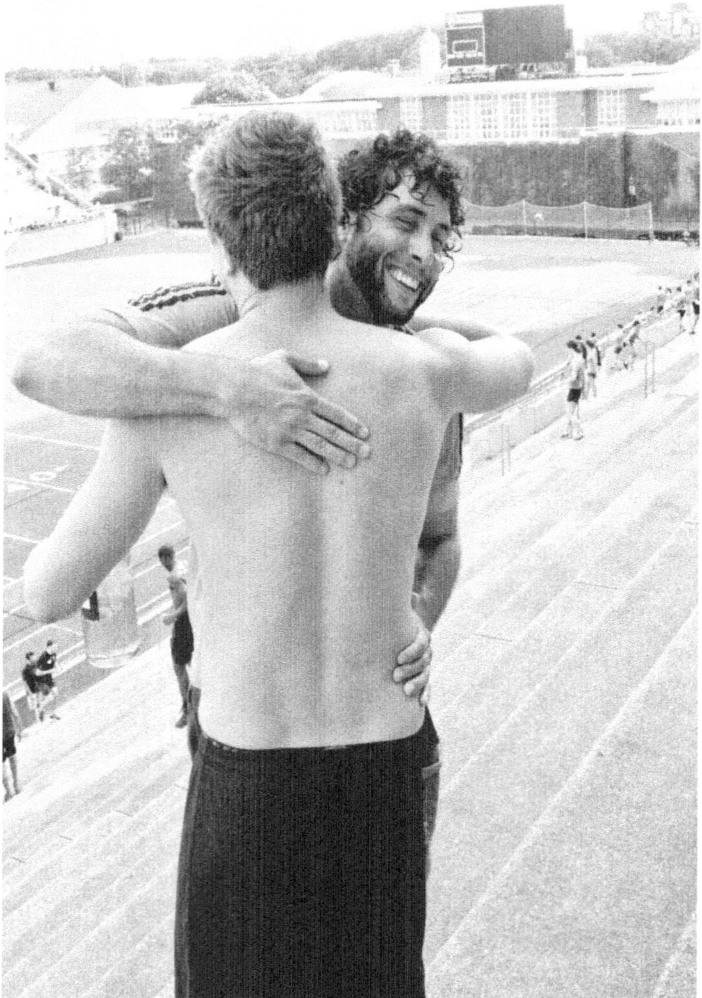

Final Thoughts

> It's the single most powerful influence that I've had in my life. On pretty much every level.
>
> —Emily Saul, November Project Boston coleader, 2016

This statement by Boston coleader Emily Saul really sums up what November Project is doing: changing the world and kicking ass. They are not only bringing fitness and positivity to local communities but also changing people's lives, which was outlined in the astoundingly personal and praising statements my survey respondents made. Members aren't just running with a group of people, they are part of something much bigger

"Working out harder and more frequently makes me a better athlete. Having friends makes me a happier, better person." I believe this statement from one of my survey participants truly sums up the way in which free fitness can change lives. Yes, you are going to work out more, probably lose a few pounds, and be able to run faster than you did before. But the real way in which it is having an impact on people's lives is through the latter part of that statement. Movements like November Project support and encourage positivity and community, through which you can become more confident, happier, stronger, and even form some of the most important relationships in your life, ultimately making you a better person.

I used to think that fitness and exercise meant going to a spin class, talking to no one, and sweating a bit before getting in my car and going home. But I have discovered that it is so much more than that. It doesn't have to be a solo activity that you resent doing just so you can order pizza for dinner, but instead it can become part of your social life. It can be something that keeps you not only physically healthy but also mentally healthy. It can be the best part of your day.

Fitness can change your life, and grassroots movements like November Project that encourage you to not only explore your city but also to get fit with others are doing just that. I hope that movements like this continue and spread across the globe, as nothing but good can come from people getting fit, making friends, and establishing a community all before seven in the morning.

So go on, what's stopping you now?

Go and find some free fitness wherever you are—who knows, maybe it could change your life.

What Happened Next

After I wrote this book, this happened to me.

May 11, 2016, 7:30 a.m.

Just Show Up

This morning started like any other November Project morning. My friend, Sarah, collected me, and we headed along to the 5:30 a.m. group. We had our usual bounce, today accompanied by an incredibly out-of-time slow clap, and then we went on to do a workout called "boroughs." This is when the stadium is divided into seven sections, or boroughs, if you will. You must do five sections over and over again, but the main goal is to get to know all the people in your boroughs, your neighbors.

Six or Not Six

I was in borough six today, and I'm not being biased when I say this, but we were the best borough. OK, maybe not the best, but we were the fucking loudest. We cheered, cursed, chanted, and smack-talked our way through thirty sections. I was elected mayor of the borough, even though I am a foreigner and have only a liquor license (suck it, Donald Trump). I loved this morning's workout: the sun was shining, awesome people surrounded me, and my borough was kicking ass. I thought this day couldn't get much better, and it was only 6:15 a.m.—boy, was I wrong.

I decided to stick around for the 6:30 group, not so I could work out again but mainly so I could chat with all my friends and catch up with people. Also, I'm Scottish, and we don't see the sun very much, so I think I just couldn't bring myself to go inside.

The Opposite of a Walk of Shame

As we sat down for the photo, I placed myself at the back. I had already been in the 5:30 photo, so it was not really fair to go front and center. There were the usual happy birthdays and announcements about the upcoming week, and then our coleaders brought out the Positivity Award. I'm going to be honest: I was not paying attention to the beginning of Emily's speech, and then I started to be more aware of what she was saying about someone who is here for a limited time. In my head I thought, *Oh, someone's like me and has to leave. We should talk.* Then all of sudden, I started to see the people around me taking out their phones, and more and more people were turning around and smiling at me. I thought, *No, don't be silly. It will be someone who is awesome. It isn't me.* Then Emily said the line, "She was one of two new people on her first workout, and they had the same name—Kathleen." All I could think was *Fuck, why did I sit so far back?* I couldn't believe it. It took some time to get to the front, so long that let's just say if I was on an awards show, then they would have had to loop the music. Once I made it to the front, I grabbed Emily and got a massive hug. And to be honest, the rest was a little bit of a blur. I was just so shocked.

On my first Wednesday at November Project over a year ago, I saw someone win the PA, and from that moment, I wanted to win it too. But I never thought I would, as the people who have won it have been some of the most amazing human beings I have ever met, and everyone knows them. They all had this presence. I know it's just an old rowing oar, but it means so much more than that. For me, November Project has changed my life by giving me a support network, changing my mind-set to be more positive, increasing my fitness to allow me to do a half marathon, and making me a happier person in myself and in life. I don't think I would have felt so at home in Boston if it hadn't been for November Project. For all of this, I will be truly grateful. Therefore, to be awarded the PA means to me that even though I am moving back to Scotland in two weeks, I am a part of this crazy November Project family. I'm going to be honest—I'm struggling to put how I feel into words.

To all my November Project people, I fucking love you all.

Resources

Boston Magazine. "November Project Shovels Summit Ave." Melissa Malamut. January 6, 2014. http://www.bostonmagazine.com/health/blog/2014/01/06/november-project-shoveling/.

Dooster Films. "November Project Summit (Madison, WI) - Part 3." Dylan Ladds. September 25, 2014. https://www.youtube.com/watch?v=eGOSOXuxLVs.

New Balance. "New Balance: November Project - The Story Behind the Movement." Kiren Aditham. July 11, 2011. https://www.youtube.com/watch?v=i5tUQzIMs3c.

Outside Magazine. "Boston's Fitness Flash Mob." Madison Kahn. May 6, 2013. http://www.outsideonline.com/1869901/bostons-fitness-flash-mob.

Runner's World. "Hugs, Sweat & Cheers." Caleb Daniloff. November 8, 2013. http://www.runnersworld.com/runners-stories/hugs-sweat-cheers.

TEDx Talks. "How to Start a Movement | November Project | TEDxBeaconStreet." December 19, 2014. https://www.youtube.com/watch?v=pAuBzKNoMEE#t=170.

Further Reading

November Project: The Book by Brogan Graham and Bojan Mandaric with Caleb Daniloff.

November Project website: http://november-project.com/

F#@k Skinny by Laura J. Ingalls

If you want to join November Project, it's really simple: find your nearest tribe and just show up. I know you won't regret it.

Acknowledgments

To every one of the crazy, badass people at November Project, you all changed my life, and without you, this project would not have been possible. At every stage, you were there willing and wanting to help me, whether it was through e-mailing me articles, filling out surveys, or just giving me a sweaty hug when I needed it most. A special thank you to Sarah, Elin, Kelly, Joey, Laura, Danimal, Erica, Selena, and of course, Emily, Chris, and Chris for contributing to this book.

Thank you to my fantastic designer, Kristen Mann, and photographer, Diana Hunt.

A huge thank-you to my professors at Northeastern University, Carl Zangler and Patty Goodman, for your enthusiasm, wisdom, and support.

Thank you to all my friends, especially Karen, for your encouragement, support, and excitement from day one. And of course, I cannot forget my mum and dad—the greatest and most successful people I know. Without them, I would not have the motivation and passion I do. Thank you for being there every step of the way.

About the Author

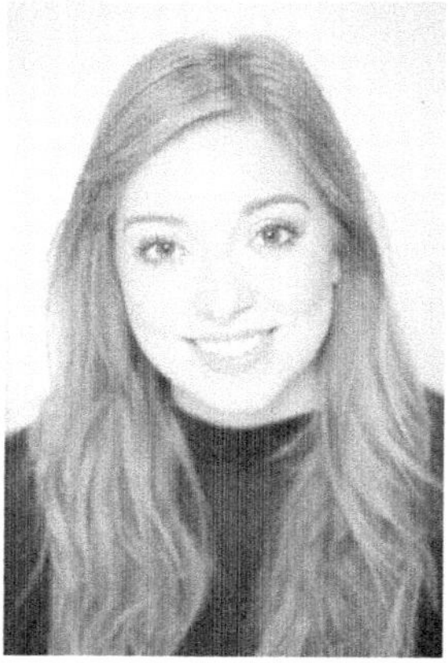

Kathleen Anderson was born in Glasgow, Scotland. She has an MSc in Corporate and Organizational Communications from Northeastern University, Boston where she spent eighteen months studying. It was during that time that she started this research and that fitness became a significant aspect of her life, which prompted her to take the leap to write her first book in the hope of inspiring others. Kathleen also has a BA in Film, Media and Marketing which she obtained at Stirling University, Scotland. She now lives in Edinburgh and writes a fitness and lifestyle blog about fitness crazes in the UK.